Lifestyles of the Trim & Healthy

MATTHEW BENNETT

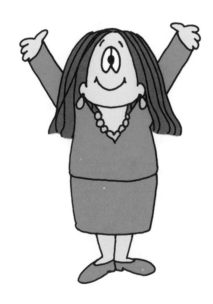

BTDT ENTERPRISES, INC.

BTDT Enterprises, Inc.
421 S. Beverly Drive, Suite 701
Beverly HIlls, CA 90212
(310) 772-7744

Printed in the USA.

ISBN: 0-9629502-9-7

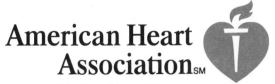
The mission of the American Heart Association is to reduce disability and death from cardiovascular diseases and stroke.

Call the American Heart Association at 1-800-AHA-USA1 (1-800-242-8721) for information on a wide range of heart health topics including exercise, high blood pressure and cholesterol prevention, dieting, quitting smoking and cardiovascular disease support groups.

Introduction

When Cathy, America's most lovable cartoon lady, first considered the idea of helping others learn about the benefits of improving their exercise and eating habits, she responded with a very predictable, "AACK!" However, once she saw how simple and effective Lifestyles of the Trim and Healthy really was, she let out a much welcome, "AHHH!"

Lifestyles of the Trim and Healthy helps lessen the stress and overwhelming feelings which often come along with getting one's life on a healthier path. Lifestyles of the Trim and Healthy offers easy-to-follow advice, tips, and strategies which have earned the approval of nationally renowned fitness experts. Delightful illustrations and motivating messages will inspire you to learn and grow, while you track your progress in the daily diary spaces.

This book provides basic nutritional and fitness information in an enjoyable, readable format so everyone can join in the fun! This book is intended to be used as a stepping stone to help you explore new areas and stimulate curiosity. Use your own experiences and common sense to get the most from this journal, and always consult with your physician before making major changes in your diet, or starting an exercise program.

Enjoy!

--Matthew Bennett

Special thanks to the following friends and supporters:

Maggie "Everything Will Be Perfect" Chun, Peter Young, Ruthie Berman, and Breck "Chock Mhool" Wilson (artists extraordinaire), Susan Valero (for believing), Dr. Betty T. Bennett (for a lifetime of inspiration and great Scrabble matches), Bob Karch (for exceptional vision), Steve Dunn (for telling me to do it myself), Mark Sisson, Lydia Puhak, and Lynn Hejtmanek (for the read), Rich Pilla (for telling me not to be a wimp), Ramona Cox (for teaching me that 18 hours is not a long work day), and of course to Cathy Guisewite (for just being Cathy).

How To Use Your Weekly Journal
(Found In The Back Of This Book)

ICONS

The four icons (or symbols) to the left of each daily journal space are provided to help you keep track of your eating and exercise patterns. Next to every symbol is an empty space in which you either fill in a check or a number as shown below:

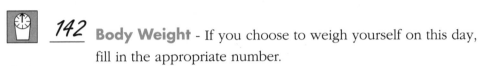 **142** **Body Weight** - If you choose to weigh yourself on this day, fill in the appropriate number.

8 **Meals** - Rate yourself on a scale of 1 to 10 (ten being the best) on how healthy your meals were.

✓ **Weight Training** - Check here if you did resistance training to strengthen your muscles.

✓ **Endurance Training** - Check here if you did cardiovascular training to strengthen your heart and lungs.

JOURNAL SPACE

Fill in the current date and use the writing space provided to remember events and deep track of your progress and achievements (see sample):

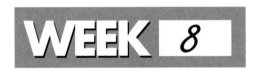 **WEEK** *8*

MONDAY

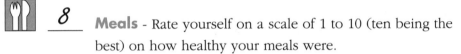 **132** *date:* 7/ 16 / 94 *notes:* *Ran an extra mile today with Devon.*
6 *Borrow yoga book from Tracy. Get babysitter for Wednesday.*
✓

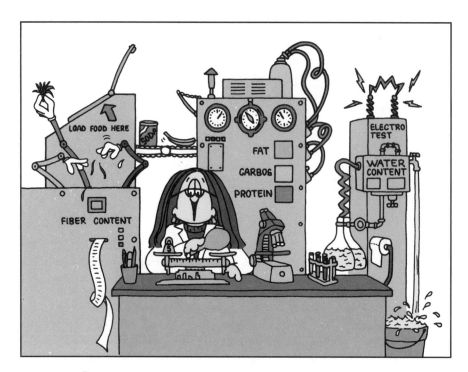

what's in what you eat

There are hundreds of differing theories on food combining, vitamin balancing, and finding the perfect meal plan, and we're going to examine every single one of them. Just kidding. For practical purposes, we will break the subject of diet into what's on your plate, and what's in what's on your plate.

The American Heart Association has developed a food guide pyramid that is broken into five levels and outlines their suggestions for maintaining a balanced diet. At the pyramid's bottom, the largest portion, we find grains, breads, cereal, rice, and pasta (6 or more daily servings recommended [DSR]). At level two, we find vegetables and fruits (5 or more DSR). Level three contains no-fat and low fat dairy products (2 to 4 DSR). Level four has lean meat, poultry, and fish, (less than 6 oz daily). Finally, the smallest top section is occupied by fats, oils, and sweets (use sparingly).

Let's define a few terms before going on:

Complex carbohydrates - Our primary and most efficient energy source, this group includes pasta, breads, grains, fruits and vegetables (usually in an unrefined form). These foods supply a wide variety of vitamins and minerals, provide all of our dietary fiber, and help to stabilize blood sugars.

Simple carbohydrate - This processed food form, commonly known as sugar, lacks vitamins, minerals and fiber. While useful as a sweetener and a preservative, it offers no nutritive value and large amounts may wreck havoc with blood sugar levels.

Protein - Found in both animal and vegetable forms, and made up of amino acids, protein plays a key role in the growth, repair and maintenance of body tissues.

Fat - See section on Fat Blasting

Calcium - Found throughout the body, but mostly in bones and teeth, calcium aids in maintaining your body's metabolism and calming nerves. While many people accept dairy products as their main supplier of this essential mineral, foods such as tofu, sardines, and dark green vegetables are also excellent sources.

Fiber - Made up of the indigestible parts of vegetables, fruits, and grains, fiber greatly assists in digestion and the body's elimination of waste products. Foods high in fiber leave you feeling satisfied and full for a long time.

When you break the food pyramid down by calories, your healthy diet consists of approximately 55-60% complex carbohydrates (4 calories per gram), less than 30% fats (9 calories per gram), and 15-20% proteins (4 calories per gram).

FDA & RDA

The U.S. Food and Drug Administration (FDA) has set minimal standards for the identification of packaged foods, and requires that if a product boasts a nutritional claim or has been fortified, then specific labeling must be provided. The label accounts for calories, protein, fat, carbohydrates, sodium, and percentages of the U.S. Recommended Daily Allowance (RDA) of protein and several specified vitamins and minerals.

The RDAs, which are updated every four to six years, are only estimates based on an "average" U.S. citizen within a segmented group (e.g., adults, children, or pregnant women) and do not cater to the special needs of individuals. However, by eating well-balanced meals and snacks (and taking a high-quality vitamin/mineral supplement, if desired), the vast majority of people will easily meet or exceed their RDAs.

Fast Fact

EATING FORTY-ONE BOWLS OF REGULAR CORN FLAKES WOULD PROVIDE YOUR BODY WITH JUST TEN GRAMS OF DIETARY FIBER.

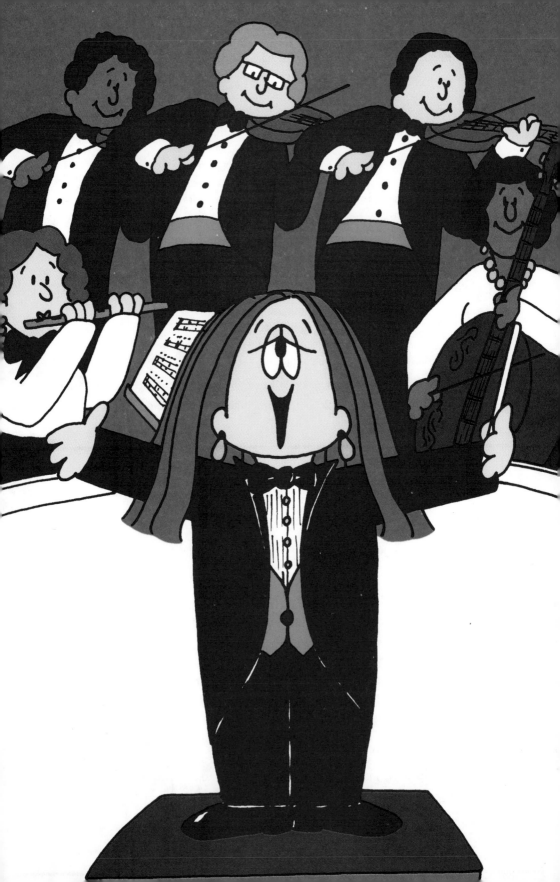

The person who says it can't

be done, should not interrupt

the person doing it.

- Chinese Proverb

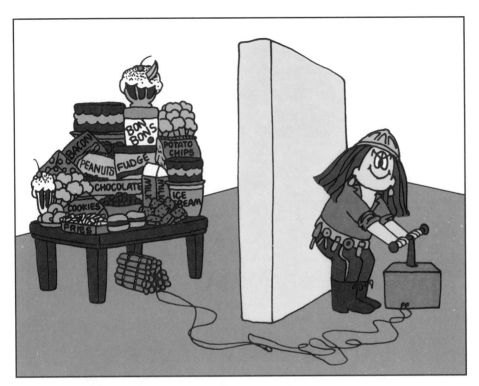

fatBlasting

WE HAVE FOUND THE ENEMY, AND IT IS FAT!

Excessive dietary fat intake has been linked to a remarkable variety of bodily ills, including: heart disease, obesity, diabetes, several types of cancer, stroke, gout, gallbladder disease, and numerous others. A gram of fat has more than double the calories of carbohydrates or protein, and excess calories convert to body fat. The truly frightening thing is, some people get more than 50% of their daily calories from fat, as opposed to a healthy 25%.

At this point, people typically ask, "But, doesn't my body need fat?" The answer is yes. Fat cushions your joints and organs, helps regulate your temperature, carries vitamins A, D, E and K, and is a high-calorie food source. In fact, all of the cells in your body contain fat. However, almost every food you eat has some amount of fat in it, and it would be almost impossible to develop a deficiency.

> ## *Fast Fact*
> CERTAIN EGG
> SUBSTITUTES
> CONTAIN MORE
> FAT THAN
> REAL EGGS.

Saturated Fats • These fats are usually found in animal products and typically remain solid at room temperature (i.e., butter and lard). Saturated fats raise blood cholesterol and are generally considered to be the least healthful source of dietary fat. Examples of foods that are particularly high in saturated fats include: high fat dairy products, many meats, chocolate, coconut, palm and palm kernel oil products.

Polyunsaturated Fats • These oils will not solidify at room temperature, or even when refrigerated. While research has indicated that these fats may help reduce blood cholesterol levels, very high intakes may be unsafe and have been connected with certain serious diseases. Examples of foods that are particularly high in polyunsaturated fats include: mayonnaise, wheat germ, margarine, canola oil, corn oil, safflower oil, and walnuts.

Monounsaturated Fats • These fats, which come from vegetable sources, are liquid at room temperature, but partially solidify when refrigerated. Monounsaturated fats may also aid in reducing cholesterol levels. Examples of foods that are high in monounsaturated fats include: canola oil, olive oil, soybean oil, shortening made from vegetable fat, and most nuts.

When reading labels to identify fats in your foods, look for the following ingredients: high fat dairy products, animal fats, any hydrogenated fat or oil, vegetable fat or oil, shortening, margarine, oil, and/or fat. While these substances do provide an extremely dense and long-lasting energy supply, the "average" person's diet is much too rich in all types of fat, and should definitely be reduced.

·········· SCRATCH THE FAT ··········

The list below offers ideas on how to cut down on the fats you eat:

1 Select lean meats, poultry and fish. Trim excess fat and remove skin whenever possible, and enjoy smaller portions (3-4 ounces).

2 Choose low fat or nonfat dairy products, and replace butter/margarine with alternate kinds of spreads and seasonings.

3 Limit egg yolks to three to four per week (use egg whites as you like).

4 Try broiling, roasting, baking or grilling meats, poultry and fish. Drain and throw away the fat that accumulates. Limit fried foods.

5 Watch out for salad dressings, nondairy creamers, and "innocent looking" desserts.

6 Use whole-grain flours.

Fast Fact

MARGARINE AND
VEGETABLE OILS
HAVE AS MANY
CALORIES AS BUTTER.

Fit Tip

GET YOURSELF A
"FAT COUNTER"
BOOK.

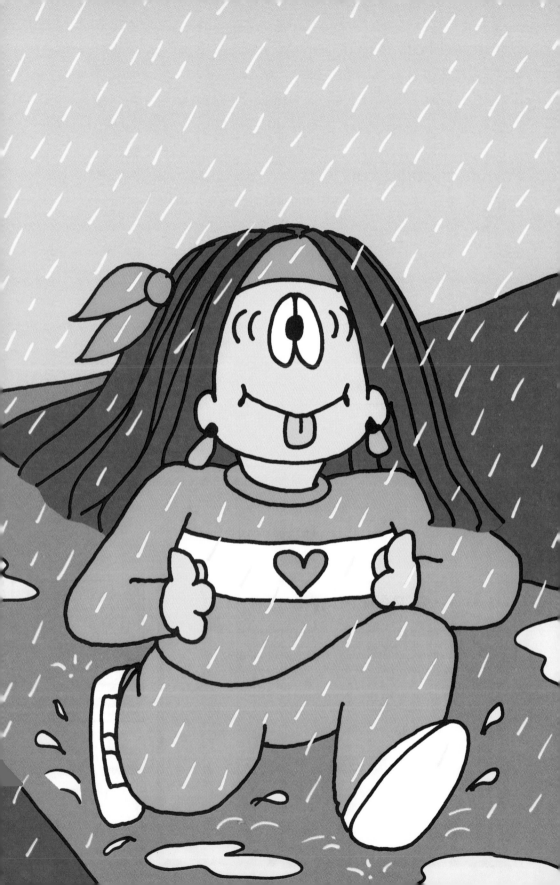

We do not always like what is

best for us in this world.

- Eleanor Roosevelt

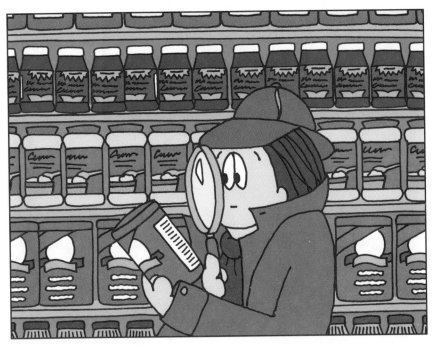

speaking Labelese

Want to better understand the nutritional value of what you consume, and avoid unpleasant surprises by profit-hungry food manufacturers? Then you need to learn to speak "labelese." A product described as, "all natural, low sodium, low fat and pure" could be anything from a skinless chicken breast to a cube of sugar to hemlock (a poisonous herb).

Fortunately, nutrition labeling has never been so well regulated. As of May, 1994, the Nutrition Labeling and Education Act (NLEA) goes into effect for all Food and Drug Related products. Before, labels could be extremely deceptive in their use of terms like, "natural," "fortified," or "improved." Now uniform definitions for terms such as these have been established. For more information, call the American Heart Association's toll-free number at 1-800-242-8721 to request a free copy of the pamphlet, "How To Read The New Food Label."

Product ingredients must be listed in descending order by weight, so closely examine the first five items in any product...do they include fats, sugars, or chemical additives? Stick with the least refined foods available in their most natural forms. Heavily fortified and/or enriched foods have often had their original nutritional value stripped out by processing. In fact, as unbelievable as it may seem, there are quite a few prepackaged "diet meals" that get over half of their calories from fat!

Fats can be especially tough to keep tabs on. Even low fat milk which is only 2% fat by weight, gets a full 30% of its calories from fat. Labels give the amount of fat per serving and list the calories from fat, so read carefully. Review "Fat Blasting" for information on the differences between hydrogenated, monounsaturated, polyunsaturated, and saturated fats that can show up in various forms (e.g., margarine, shortenings, lard, oils).

Aim to reduce the percentage of fats in the foods you consume to 30% or lower. Make dietary changes one step at a time and don't try to change lifelong eating habits overnight. Reducing your total fat intake will automatically help you achieve your healthy diet goals — simply eating well-balanced meals that are low in sugar and fats, and high in carbohydrates and fiber.

THE fat OF THE LAND

Fat-free - Contains insignificant amounts of fat, less than 0.5 g per serving.

Low fat - 3 g or less per serving.

Low in saturated fat - No more than 1 g of saturated fat and no more than 15% calories from saturated fat.

Low in cholesterol - No more than 20 mg cholesterol per serving and no more than 2 g saturated fat.

Lean - Refers to fat content of meat, poultry, seafood, and game meats. Less than 10 g fat, less than 4.5 g saturated fat, and less than 95 mg cholesterol per serving and per 100 g.

Extra-lean - Less than 5 g fat, less than 2 g saturated fat, and less than 95 mg cholesterol per serving and per 100 g.

Reduced/less fat - 25% less fat than regular version of that product. If reference food already qualifies as a "low" product, lighter version cannot use term reduced.

Light - One third fewer calories or 50% less fat than regular version of the food. If food gets 50% or more of its calories from fat, reduction must be 50% of the fat. Light can also describe texture and color as long as it is explained as such on the label.

Percent fat-free - Must be low fat/fat-free product and must refer to amount of fat present in 100 g of the food.

Modified fat - Must state how modified from regular product; for example, "modified fat cheesecake contains 35% less fat than our regular cheesecake."

Fit Tip

FROZEN YOGURT HAS ABOUT HALF THE NUTRIENTS OF REGULAR YOGURT.

Information courtesy of the Food and Drug Administration.

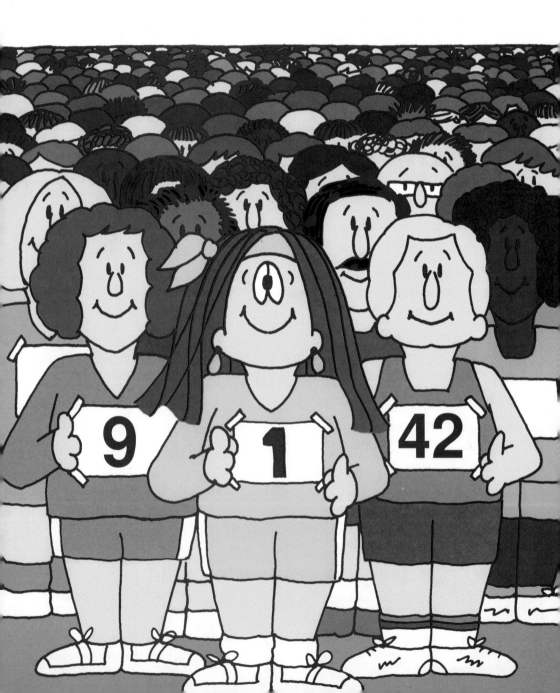

One who has begun the task

has half done it.

- Horace

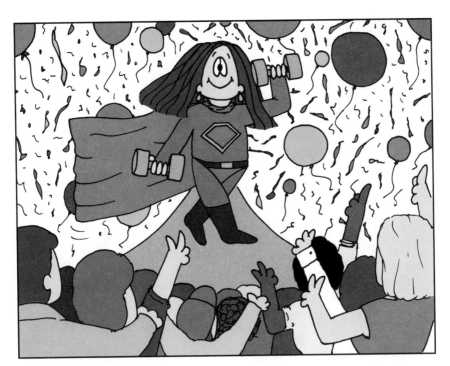

why exercise?

"Can I become a gourmet chef without ever going into my kitchen?"
"Can I drive my car from New York to California without stopping to refuel?"
"Can I lose weight and maintain a healthier lifestyle without exercising?"

The questions above can all be answered the same way, "Nice idea, but don't be silly." When you lose pounds by depriving yourself of calories or loading up on high-protein foods, the weight dropped comes mostly from a loss of water and muscle tissue. Your body reacts to this temporary "starvation" by conserving energy and storing fat. Eventually, you will gain back the pounds and have to deal with additional new fat reserves. People on "popular" diets who have body fat percentage tests, often find that they have increased their ratio of body fat even if they have lost weight!

If you want to keep the weight off and feel physically fit, you have to exercise. Most people never think about it, but it's primarily your muscles that burn up the calories you consume; fat, bone and skin just sit there. Exercised muscles respond by becoming stronger and leaner, and the more lean muscle mass you have, the more calories you will use up all day long.

Fast Fact

EXERCISE IS ONE OF THE WORLD'S GREATEST STRESS RELIEVERS.

Regular physical activity provides so many super benefits it would take pages to list them all, but here's a sample:

Strengthens your heart and improves circulation • Your heart is a muscle, and physical activity will help it to pump more blood with less effort.

Helps maintain your ideal weight • Exercising quickens your metabolism, so even after a workout, your body continues to use more fuel for a period of time.

Helps fight stress and mental fatigue • People who train regularly are more relaxed and cope better with depression than their inactive counterparts.

Improves digestion and may reduce your appetite • Food will pass through you faster, plus many people don't eat as much when they exercise.

Tones muscles, encourages good posture, and controls your weight • Nothing compares to regular physical activity for developing lean, strong, fat-burning muscles.

Gives you an overall sense of sound health • Exercise makes you look and feel better, increases your energy level and stamina, and gives you that positive boost to help you deal with everyday life!

Exercise can become a valued (and even enjoyable) part of your life if you take the right approach. Carefully study all of the exercise information presented for helpful hints for getting started and sticking with it.

GETTING STARTED

Designing a rewarding exercise program for yourself takes a certain amount of planning. To ensure positive results, you should:

1 Set specific, realistic goals - Write down exactly what you would like to achieve in the long and short term. Be kind and go easy at first, always rewarding yourself for special accomplishments.

2 Plan your regular exercise time - Set a specific activity period and stay with it. If you "wait for the best time to fit it in," it might never happen.

3 Track your achievements - Keep a written progress record...you'll be amazed at your changes over time.

4 Select the activities that you enjoy most - Some people enjoy revisiting sports/play from their past, while others prefer the challenge of a new endeavor.

5 Consult with an "expert" - Speak with someone who enjoys exercising and tap into their ideas and resources.

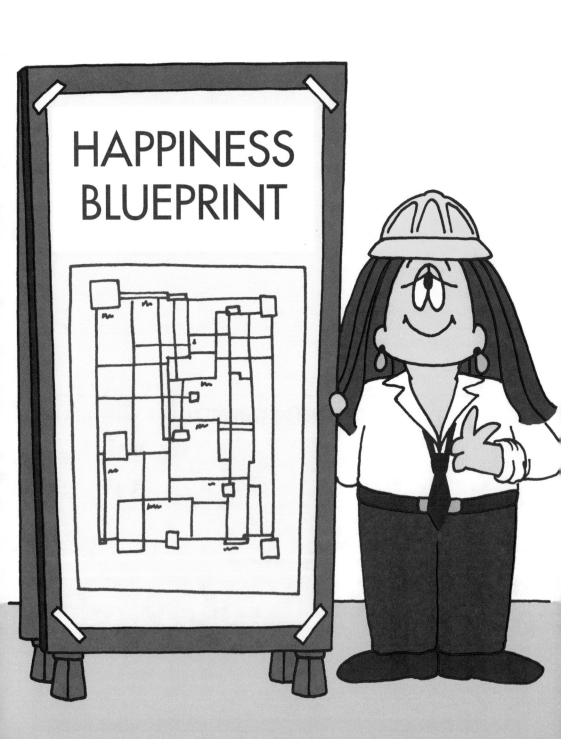

Whatever you can do or dream
you can, begin it. Boldness has
genius, magic and power in it.
Begin it now.

- Goethe

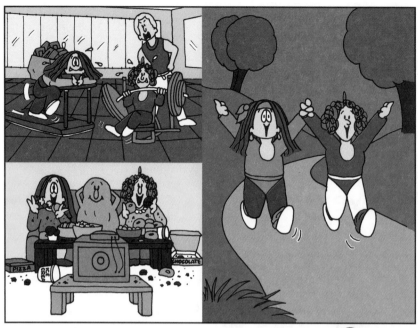

too much
too little

two fit

Starting an exercise program can be pretty intimidating. "How often do I have to work-out?" "For how long?" "How hard must I train to see real results?" These questions confuse many beginners so much, they never get started at all. The good news is that once you understand a few simple ideas, you can easily address these issues.

First, let's break exercise into to the broad areas of aerobic (or cardiovascular) training and resistance training. Aerobic activities (e.g., walking, running, rope jumping, etc.): 1) Burn fat as they benefit your heart and lungs; 2) Almost always use your legs; 3) Last at least twenty minutes; and 4) Should be performed at a comfortable pace.

The FIT formula below establishes several basic guidelines to follow:

Frequency - Schedule exercise at least three times per week.

Intensity - Keep your heart beating within a range of 65-80% of your maximum heart rate per minute (220 minus your age = your maximum). If you are 35 years old, your target range would be 120-148 heart beats per minute (220 minus 35 = 185 / 185 times .65 = 120 / 185 times .80 = 148). You should be breathing deeply, but not huffing and puffing (keep a pace at which you can carry on a conversation).

Time - Each session should last a minimum of 15 to 20 minutes.

Start slowly and work your way up. If you take it too easy (staying below your range), you won't burn much fat. If you push too hard (exceeding your range), your body will actually decrease the amount of fat it's burning. In the beginning, you may be amazed how little movement it takes to bring you into your target range. As your fitness improves, however, you will be able to do more and more.

Resistance training (e.g., weightlifting, push-ups, sit-ups, etc.) firms and tones your muscles. While excellent for shaping and building strength, resistance exercises do not directly burn body fat. However, by maintaining or increasing your lean body mass, you become a more efficient calorie/fat burner, and that's the goal of everyone who works out.

Ideally, find an instructor or knowledgeable friend to guide you and correct your form through your early exercise sessions (especially for resistance training). Whether you do or not, here are some helpful pointers to get you started: 1) Concentrate on your movements and breathe deeply, exhaling during exertion; 2) Don't work the same muscle group two days in a row; 3) Pick up an exercise book and spend a few hours studying it; 4) Select weights and movements you can control; and 5) Lifting heavy weights for limited repetitions (4-6 reps) tends to build size, while working with light weights (10-12 reps) is better for toning and firming.

Warming Up To The Idea

Warming up before exercising and stretching afterwards are two of the most important things you can do to prevent sports injuries, yet far too many people neglect these activities. The point of warming up is to increase your blood circulation and prepare your muscles and joints for action. While any exercise book/video will explain many movements that can help you accomplish this, one of the best methods is to simply go through the motions of your exercise or sport at half speed until you naturally loosen up (five to ten minutes is usually enough time, although people who work out in the morning sometimes require a bit more).

Proper stretching helps keep your whole body feeling strong, improves your posture, and decreases sprains and strains. Whatever movements you choose, remember that stretching should feel good; keep it comfortable and never stretch to the point of pain. Move slowly, without bouncing, and hold each position for at least thirty seconds. Always stretch after warming up or exercising...stretching cold muscles can actually do more harm than good.

Fit Tip

THERE ARE MANY EXCELLENT EXERCISE VIDEOS AND TV PROGRAMS TO HELP YOU GET FIT.

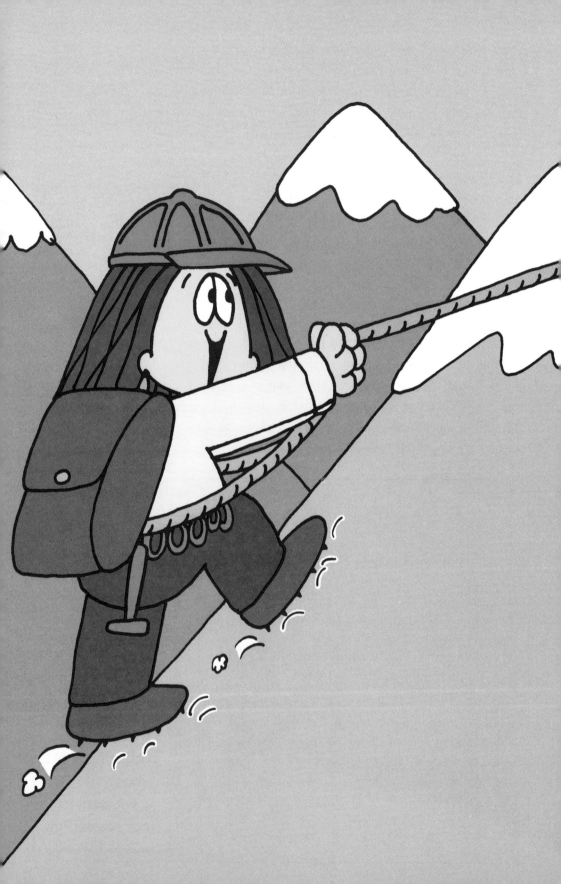

It is not because things are difficult that we do not dare; it is because we do not dare that they are difficult.

- Seneca

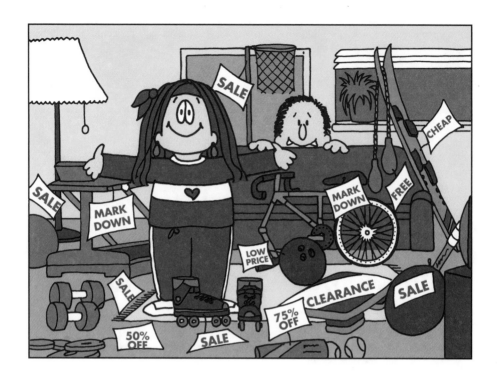

rejoice in **choice**

So many activities, so little time! The list of sports and exercises you can enjoy is practically endless, and each has its own advantages and appeal. In fact, choosing several different forms of exercise to develop a wider variety of body parts and better muscle balance (called "cross-training") has become one of the most popular and beneficial techniques people use to create a program that's just right for them. It also helps keep one from falling into an exercise rut! The following brief descriptions will get you on the right track:

Running/Jogging - This popular calorie-burner strengthens your heart and
lungs while improving overall muscle tone. To get started, all you need is a good pair of running shoes and a comfortable outfit (women should strongly consider investing in a quality athletic bra). Try to avoid concrete or other "unforgiving" surfaces and make sure you drink enough fluids.

Walking - This low-cost, no-hassle winner has become
the first choice of exercise enthusiasts all over the world. Offering the same advantages as jogging, walking is easier on the body and perfect for a beginner's program. Just make sure you are moving fast enough to keep your heart beating in its target range.

> **Fast Fact**
> RESEARCH SHOWS THAT MORNING EXERCISERS ARE LESS LIKELY TO QUIT.

Aerobics - Millions of people have gotten hooked on this invigorating combination of calisthenics and dance. You may take classes, or experiment at home with one of the excellent videos available. Pick an appropriate pace for your fitness level (novice through advanced) and explore different styles (low-impact, water aerobics, jazz, western).

Stepping - Stair climbing/stepping is a terrific conditioner that works your body as hard as running does, but it's easier on the joints and less likely to cause injuries. Whether you use real stairs, take bench step classes, or jump on a stepping machine, you'll enjoy great benefits for your cardiovascular system and lower body.

Cycling - The exercise bike is an American classic. Indoor cycling offers results for people of all ages and fitness levels — it's easy, safe, and efficient. People enjoy outdoor cycling by touring, racing, or just pleasure riding. Keep the pedals moving constantly for the best work-out.   Budget carefully for all the costs of your bike and related gear.

Swimming - Exercising in the water strengthens your muscles, builds your heart and lungs, and involves practically no risk of injury. Perfect, right? Not quite. Contrary to what many people believe, swimming is not an efficient fat-burner. Because of a need to maintain heat and buoyancy, all bodies tend to hold on to their fat more while in the water. Regardless, swimming is still a fine choice for improving your overall fitness.

Weights - Training with barbells, dumbbells, and machines that provide resistance offers two unique advantages over other athletic activities: 1) It allows you to focus on one specific area of your body at a time, toning and shaping through concentrated movements; and 2) Weightlifting strengthens your major muscle groups, making it easier to participate in other sports. Also, remember that active muscles burn calories.

Martial Arts - These activities, which include karate, judo, boxing, and others, provide exceptional toning, strength, stretching, and coordination training. While excellent for learning self-defense and building self-confidence, there are also non-contact varieties.

Racquet sports, jumping rope, skating, hiking, skiing, and golfing are among dozens of other exciting activities that combine exercise and fun. Find your own favorites!

SELF-IMAGE

Many of us base our self-images on messages we received during our childhoods and adolescent years. While these notions may not be very accurate or flattering, they are usually quite difficult to change. One of the remarkable gifts of developing a healthier lifestyle is the positive overall effect it can have on how you feel about yourself and everything you do. Taking better care of yourself through exercise and proper nutrition, will boost both your energy and confidence levels. Be patient and good to yourself, giving old habits and perceptions the time they need to change.

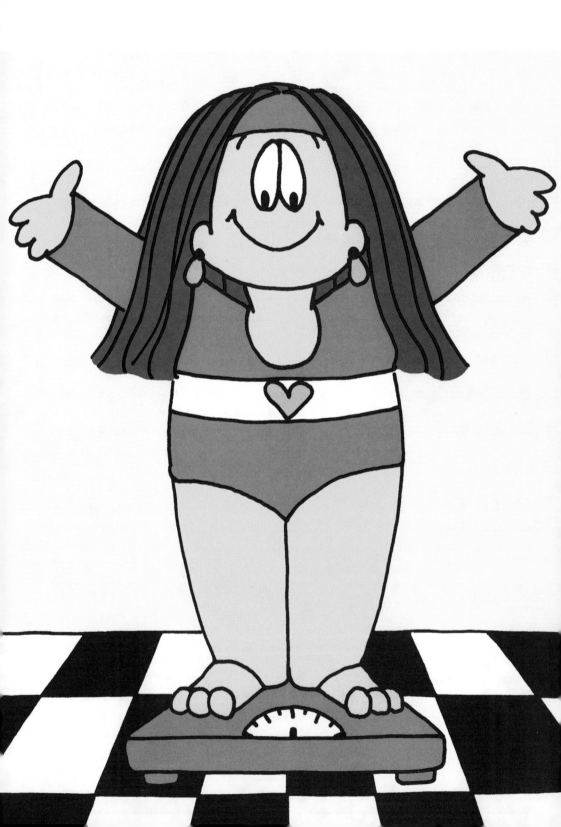

Whether you think you can or think you can't, you are right.

- Henry Ford

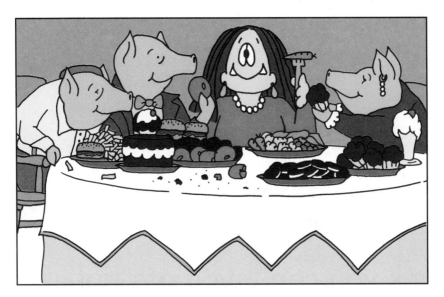

mastering your own **density**

Everyone is concerned about the environment these days. However, the environments concerning us involve saving yourself, along with the rainforest! We're talking about your eating environments. In what rooms of your home do you usually snack? What signals trigger you to "pig out?" Do you find smart restaurant dining overly challenging?

Eating cues, whether for carrot sticks or carrot cake, differ significantly from person to person. People respond to visual stimulation, scents, and even sounds when it comes to feeding themselves. The four major "zones" to address in this regard are in-home, restaurants, parties, and vacations.

In-home - How often have you reached for a sugary morsel simply because it was in front of you? When it comes to snacking, what you see is what you get, so clear the decks. If you live alone, it's time to dump the junk...out with the bad, in with the good! If you have to compromise with others, at least go through your refrigerator and your cabinets and "bury" the fattening offenders behind healthier alternatives. Enlist as much support as possible from family and/or housemates.

Restaurants - Will power and advance planning are the keys to eating smart while dining out. Always have a light snack before leaving your home, to take the edge off your hunger and help you resist forbidden temptations on the menu. Don't be embarrassed to ask your waiter to serve heavy sauces or dressings on the side, or for your meal to be prepared without butter or cheese. Remember, you're the customer, and the customer is always right.

Parties - "One more drink isn't going to kill you." "You look good the way you are." "Have some fun, it's just one night." These are the dangerous words of typical party-goers. Don't succumb to the influence of peer pressure. Think before you bite! Make thoughtful decisions based on your own needs and desires, not the opinions and taunting of others. A polite, but firm, "No, thank-you," will let others know that you have every intention of sticking to a healthy game plan. Be proud of your commitment to sound nutrition...after all, it's your well-being.

Vacations - We have just one thing to say to people who gain weight and feel bad because they use travelling as an excuse to eat poorly and shelve their exercise programs; you reap what you sow (bad pun!). Enjoy your holidays, but don't throw away your good sense. If your accommodations don't provide the best dining or work-out options, modify your routines and choices to fit the environment. As always, perfection is not the goal! Do the best you can wherever you are, and have fun. You'll find many ways to take advantage of your new energy level and active lifestyle.

The Great Weight Debate

To weigh, or not to weigh, that is the question. The answers range from programs that forbid using a scale, to those that insist on checking your personal poundage twice a day! The pro-weighers argue that since most people can't get their body fat percentage tested daily, body weight is the easiest way to keep score in the battle of the bulge. By constantly tipping the scales, you give yourself a clear goal, and you trip off an early alarm when you get off track.

Anti-weighers claim that pounds have nothing to do with fitness or health...its how you feel and look that really matter. They claim that varying bone densities, body types, water losses/gains, and the fact that muscle weighs more than fat, make the scale's readings meaningless. If how you look and feel isn't enough for you, these folks believe in the use of a tape measure and/or body fat tests to chart your progress.

If you choose to weigh yourself as part of your trim and healthy lifestyle, follow these tips: 1) For consistency, use the same good-quality scale; 2) Always weigh yourself at the same time of day, wearing clothing that you know the weight of; and 3) Don't panic if you see unexplainable, temporary set-backs. Your body goes through literally millions of reactions and changes that can affect your weight...don't let focusing on the numbers discourage you or cloud the bigger health picture.

Fit Tip

DRINK 8 EIGHT-OZ GLASSES OF WATER EVERY DAY.

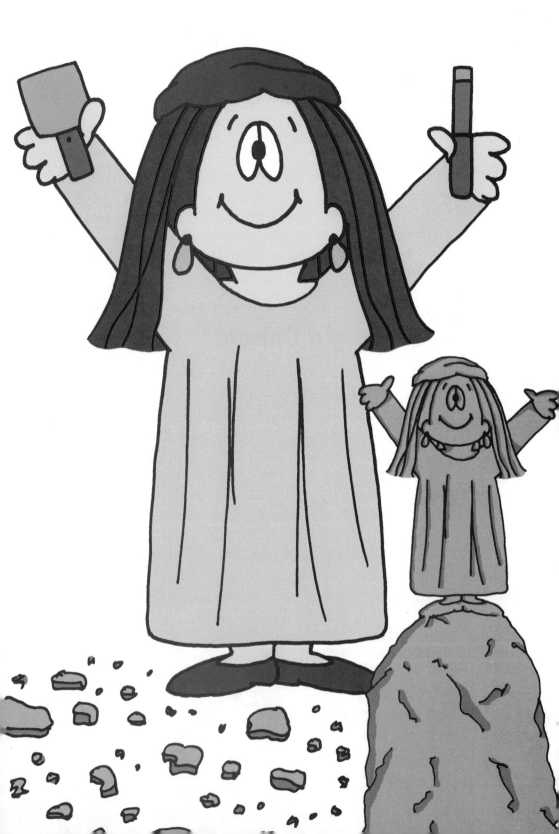

Don't compromise yourself--

you're all you've got.

- Lisa Hampton

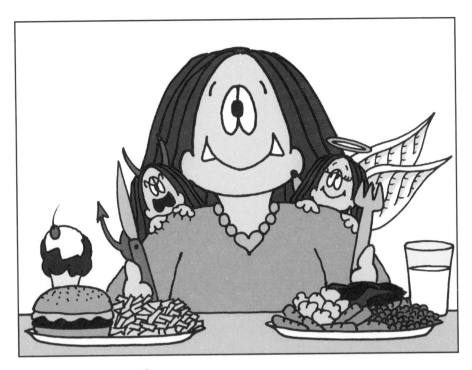

staying Stronger

"WHEN WE SEEK PERFECTION, WE SEEK FAILURE."

At first glance, the quote above seems strange. But, when you really think about it, these words carry a very important message. No person or thing in the world is perfect, and when we set unrealistic unattainable goals for ourselves, we are guaranteed to have a disappointing experience. Practice does not make perfect — practice makes for improvement. One of the biggest obstacles people face as they strive to better their eating and exercise habits is getting past slips and mistakes. Don't let missing a day of exercise or having a piece of cake become a signal that you can't make the grade. Everyone has off days, so give yourself a break. What really counts is your overall lifestyle and what you do on a consistent basis.

If someone tells you that they have discovered an effortless way to become fit and healthy, better check again. Nothing highly valuable or desirable comes without effort. Dieting or taking pills simply masks the problem temporarily. Developing a healthier lifestyle including sound nutrition and regular exercise will give you real results that last a lifetime.

WITH THESE THOUGHTS IN MIND, HERE ARE SOME TIPS ON HOW TO STAY MOTIVATED:

1 Set realistic long-term and short-term goals which pinpoint your own personal objectives. Don't let friends or family push you too far or too fast. Ultimately, positive permanent lifestyle changes have got to be made by you and for you.

2 Reward yourself every time you reach a goal, no matter how small. Whether it's a massage, new shoes, or an evening out, make sure to give yourself those well-deserved pats on the back.

3 Surround yourself with people who believe in you and what you can achieve. A team of positive supporters can be just the ticket for helping you through the more challenging times. Don't let anyone say you can't, when you know you can.

4 Enjoy a wide variety of athletic activities and foods to avoid stagnation. Explore unchartered waters to keep things stimulating.

5 Getting yourself a training partner, joining a club, or taking lessons are all terrific ways to boost motivation and meet others who share your interests.

6 Expect a certain amount of fluctuation in your weight and how you feel. Everyone gets into slumps at times; changing your routine around or taking a couple of days off can be very refreshing.

7 Study exercise and nutrition by reading books, experimenting with low-fat recipes, and taking classes. Become an expert and be proud of your new healthy lifestyle.

RELAXATION AND VISUALIZATION

Used by everyone from politicians to top athletes to set and reach goals, visualization helps people turn their dreams into reality. Start out by relaxing your body and mind...take a hot bath, meditate, stretch, or do whatever works for you. Get comfortable in a spot where you will not be disturbed, close your eyes, and picture yourself accomplishing your goals. See the new you, feeling terrific and looking exactly how you want to look. Take your time and be specific. Focus on every detail of your life — eating smart, exercising, working and playing — until you create a healthy, happy image. Start today, and get ready for some surprising results. Everyone (at any age) can visualize or project positive thoughts and achieve remarkable rewards by experimenting with these techniques.

Fast Fact

TUNA PACKED IN OIL HAS SEVEN TIMES MORE FAT THAN WATER-PACKED.

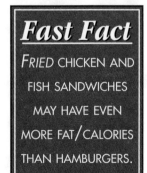

Fast Fact

FRIED CHICKEN AND FISH SANDWICHES MAY HAVE EVEN MORE FAT/CALORIES THAN HAMBURGERS.

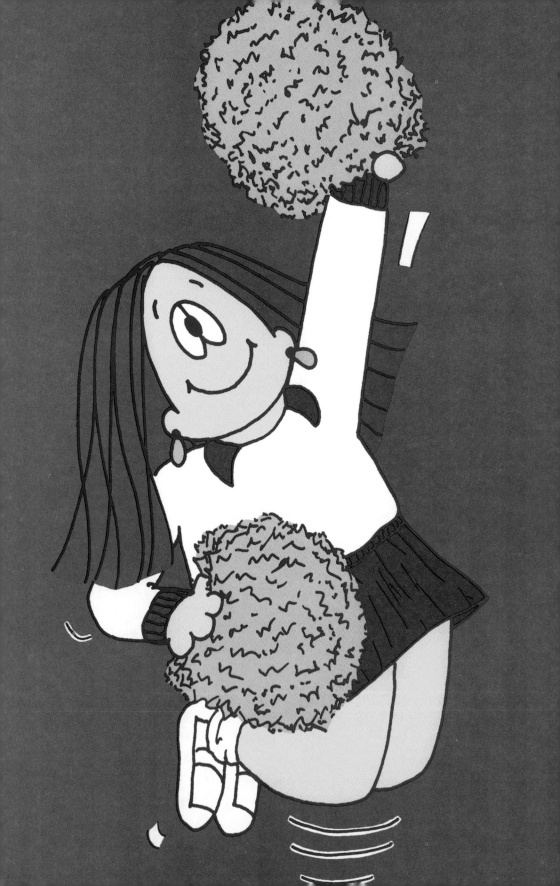

Nothing great was ever

accomplished without

enthusiasm.

- Emerson

Don't be a
yoyo

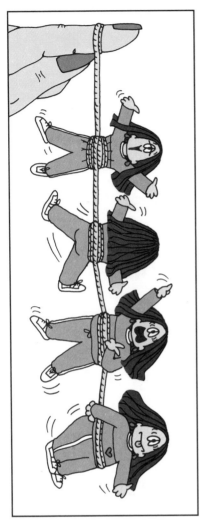

Laura goes on a high-protein, low carbohydrate diet and loses fifteen pounds in just two weeks. However, just when it seems she has found an absolute miracle, she gains back the fifteen pounds she lost plus another five for good measure (or bad measure, as the case may be!). Now desperate, Laura decides she is going to starve her body into submission by eating just one 600 calorie meal a day. At first the results look promising, but within a month she's right back where she started. Does this pattern of up and down weight loss sound familiar to you?

Brace yourself, because here is the shocking explanation to Laura's problem: **Fad diets and devices don't work!** They never have, they never will, and the only thing they're good for is taking people's money and turning them into dieting yoyos. The way to lose unwanted fat and feel good about yourself permanently is to eat smart and exercise regularly. It seems almost too simple when you see it in plain language, yet that's the whole story.

There are no magic formulas or creams, no instant herbal pills, no "secret" wraps, and no single "state-of-the-art" exerciser that will permanently remove unwanted fat from your body. All of the hype and wild claims are exactly what they look like...hype and wild claims. If there was some mystical no-effort way to actually lose fat and become healthier, why would "new and improved" diets and inventions keep popping up every week?

> ## Fit Tip
>
> **FADS ARE LIKE WAVES, UNPREDICTABLE AND ABRUPT. GOOD HABITS ARE LIKE THE TIDE, SURE AND STEADY.**

The human body is mainly made up of bone, skin, muscle, organs and fat. When you dramatically reduce your caloric intake, or fast, your body will fight to store fat and conserve energy while burning up both muscle and fat for fuel. Most people are surprised to discover that the weight lost by depriving themselves of food is actually one-third fat and two-thirds muscle.

Eventually, dieters go off their diets and quickly gain back the temporary fat and water loss along with an increase in fat-storing enzymes. Now programmed to conserve and store, the body winds up putting on more fat than ever. Depending on whether or not one does resistance exercises (e.g., weightlifting), one may never replace the lost muscle tissue. The end result is that the dieter weighs at least as much as before, with a higher percentage of body fat.

High-protein, low-carbohydrate diets tend to be high in fat and force the body to use fat as its primary fuel source. While carbohydrates burn very efficiently in your system, fats don't and they leave behind an acidic residue called ketones. As a person's concentration of ketones increases, they run the risk of developing ketosis, a dangerous blood disorder.

At best, fad diets lead to short-term weight loss based mostly on dehydration and damage to lean muscle mass, leaving users feeling listless, irritable and unsatisfied. In the worst case scenario, they lead to ketosis, high cholesterol, kidney problems and even fatalities. *To lose unwanted fat and feel good about yourself consistently, eat smart and exercise regularly.*

INCIDENTALLY...

The following questions people often ask themselves have something important in common: Should I walk a few blocks to the store or take the car? Should I ride the escalator to the next floor or use the stairs? Should I vegetate in front of the television for half of the day or go do something productive? These decisions all involve incidental exercise -- the type of physical activities a person chooses to participate in without actually working out. It's the calories you burn simply running around all day being you, and just about everyone gets some amount of incidental exercise every day.

While not a replacement for your regular exercise program, increasing activity levels even a little bit on a daily basis can provide an important first step to enjoying a trim and healthy lifestyle. The funny thing about physical activity is, the more you do, the easier it becomes to do even more! So, take a walk, take the stairs, and take a healthier new look at your life.

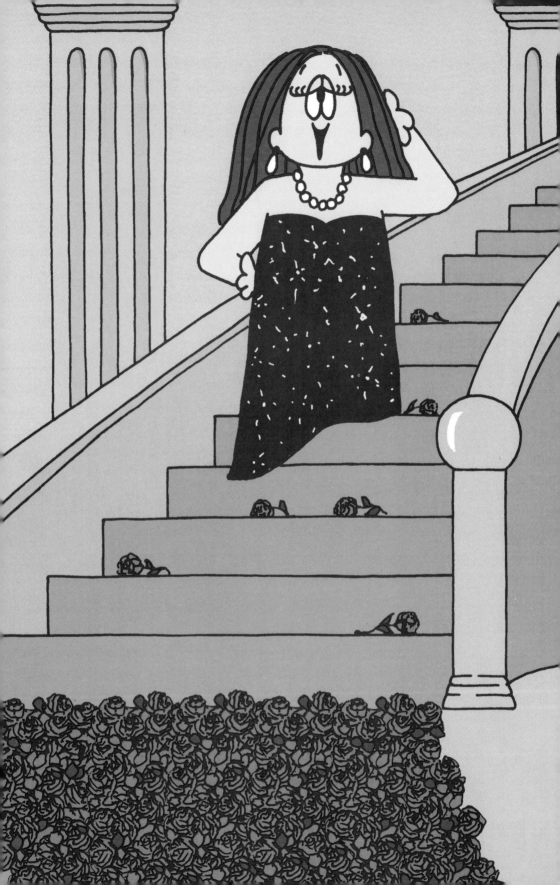

Things do not change,

we change.

- H. D. Thoreau

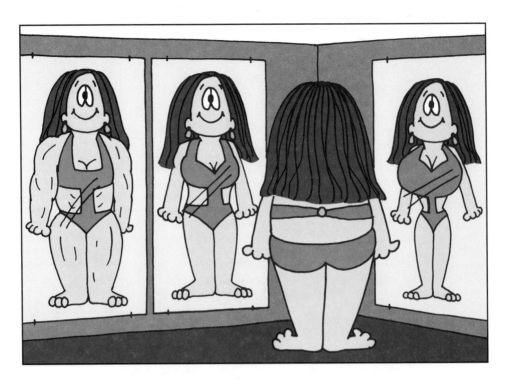

myth Busters

If you're looking for miracle thigh-reducing creams, the newest no-effort fat-burning machines, or ancient herbs guaranteed to rid the world of unsightly cellulite, you've come to the wrong place. Here are explanations of some of the most common health and fitness misconceptions:

myth #1 *If I exercise my legs and buttocks often and hard enough, I will burn off all the cellulite.*

First things first...cellulite is nothing more than plain old fat. The word "cellulite" was made up by some creative people to describe the subcutaneous (just under the skin) fat that tends to accumulate around the thighs and buttocks. Fat looks pocked or lumpy in these areas due to the texture of the skin, and has been given its own name solely for marketing purposes. You can't lose fat from just one area of the body (unless you resort to surgery). Fat exists throughout your entire system and never belongs to just one area or body part.

myth #2 *If I lift weights, I'll develop huge muscles and lose coordination.*

Everyone from professional dancers to physical therapists now recognizes the unique benefits of weightlifting; nothing achieves faster or better results when it comes to shaping the body. Of course, if you train with extremely heavy barbells doing low repetitions for two hours a day, five days a week, you will get somewhat larger and more defined (but, still not nearly as muscular as most people imagine!). Regular training with lighter weights for high repetitions will provide the firming and toning effect most people desire. And remember, it's your muscles that burn calories.

myth #3   *Exercising twice a hard will burn double the calories.*

In the words of a famous song, "It ain't necessarily so." If you consistently exercise above your target heart range, or work the same body parts too frequently, you run the risk of overtraining. Overstepping your cardiovascular limits burns up too much muscle along with the fat, as your system draws upon all available sources to supply the excessive energy demand. Even properly exercised muscles need time to recuperate and repair between workouts (especially as one gets older).

myth #4   *If I am very active during the day, and exhausted at night, I must be getting enough exercise to be healthy.*

Sorry. Your activities may burn calories and genuinely wear you out, but the proven way to strengthen your heart and improve your overall fitness level, is to raise your heart beat into its target range for at least fifteen to twenty minutes a day, three to four days a week.

VITAMINS - an easy pill to swallow

When asked why they take vitamins, people typically give the following answers: To increase energy levels, feel better, live longer, and fight off disease and illness. While consistently eating a balanced daily diet of fresh foods (including 3-5 servings of vegetables, 2-3 servings of fruit, 2-3 servings of protein, and 6-11 servings of grains) is the ideal way to get your vitamins, it's not always so easy. Today, more than ever before, physicians, dieticians, and nutritionists agree that taking a vitamin/mineral supplement every day may make good healthy sense.

In making selections, look for products that offer these quality features:

CAPSULES CONTAINING POWDER - Smaller capsules are easier to swallow, plus powders dissolve faster and are much gentler on your stomach than rock-hard tablets.

PURE, ALL NATURAL INGREDIENTS - Look for hypo-allergenic vitamins and minerals in their safest, most effective forms. Avoid artificial coloring, binders, preservatives, lubricants, and chemical additives.

NON-ACIDIC, BASIC FORMULAS - Don't choose a supplement from a manufacturer who throws in everything but the kitchen sink; herbs, pollens, roots, and the like all have their places, but not taking up space in your vitamin pill.

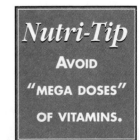

Nutri-Tip

AVOID

"MEGA DOSES"

OF VITAMINS.

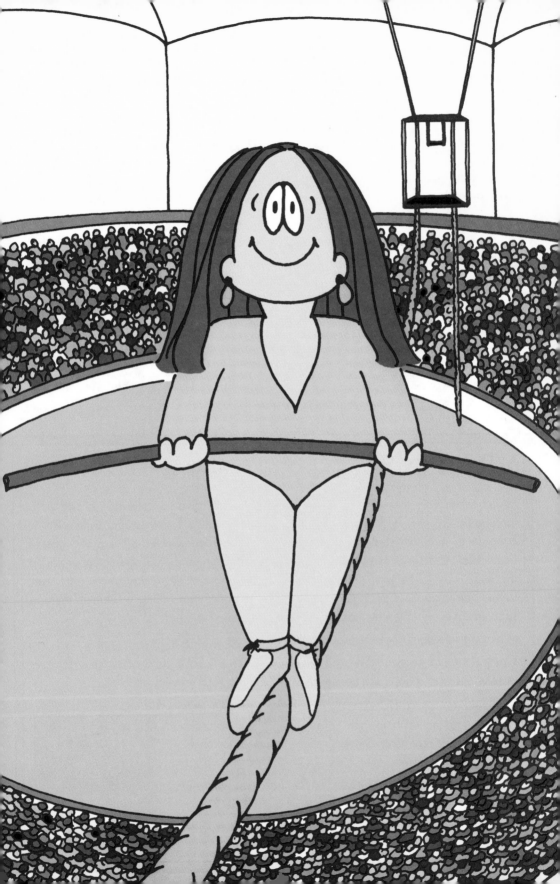

Nothing is so exhausting

as indecision, and nothing

is so futile.

- Bertrand Russell

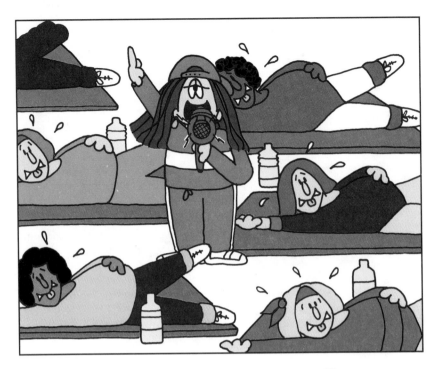

exercising for two

Years ago, pregnant women were cautioned to avoid any form of exercise more strenuous than walking. Experts now recognize that the fetus is well-cushioned in the womb and that exercise contributes to one's overall sense of well-being. Just follow a few sensible rules and you need not sacrifice your level of fitness or good health*:

- Carefully monitor your heart rate (research suggests staying under 140 beats per minute).

- Replace fluids frequently.

- Stick with exercises and sports you are accustomed to.

- Listen to your body - whether it says full steam ahead (within your target pulse range), slow down, or stop completely.

- Avoid activities that involve high impact, jumping, or any chance of falling or being struck (such as downhill skiing, horseback riding, most racquet sports, etc).

After you've done your warm-up, the safest and most beneficial exercises you can enjoy are swimming, stationary bicycling, walking, low-impact calisthenics/aerobics, and dancing. Stay aware of the frequency, duration, and intensity of your sessions and always finish with an adequate cool-down period. Many health clubs have excellent maternity exercise classes, and there are dozens of helpful books and tapes.

*A much greater degree of caution is necessary when dealing with a complicated pregnancy. Check with your careprovider regarding any exercise programs or special conditions.

GETTING BACK INTO SHAPE

Although many changes in body shape happen during pregnancy, these transformations are related to carrying a baby. Once your delivery is over, establishing a healthy pattern of exercise and nutrition will help you regain muscle tone and lose your pregnancy weight. Unfortunately, time is not on your side where regaining tone in stretched abdominal muscles and losing extra pounds is concerned. The more time passes, the worse sagging muscles will get. A well-planned, consistent exercise program will not only help you regain muscle tone and lose weight, but will also improve circulation, promote the healing of abdominal muscles, decrease swelling, relieve tension, and reduce the risk of back problems.

BEFORE YOU BEGIN ANY EXERCISE PROGRAM, CHECK WITH YOUR DOCTOR. Postpartum exercise classes are often available at local hospitals, YWCAs, or community centers. Once again, if going out is too difficult, treat ourself to an exercise videotape or book — there are plenty of good ones available. Always exercise using proper techniques and move at a pace that doesn't exhaust you. Don't reduce caloric intake drastically, especially if you are breastfeeding (nursing actually helps postpartum moms lose weight). Eating sensible, balanced meals and sticking to a comfortable exercise program will help you achieve and maintain your ideal weight faster than you think.

Work on reaching goals one at a time on a reasonable schedule. Aim for improvement, not perfection! And of course, check with your doctor before you resume exercising.

RAISING HEALTHIER CHILDREN

Childhood obesity is on the rise. Two of the notable reasons for this phenomenon may be:
1) TV, video games, and other passive activities have replaced sports and active playing.
2) The amazing assortment of fast food and junk foods available.

Today's parents need to make a special effort to help children get more excited about exercise and active recreation. The biggest influences come through providing positive role models and by direct participation in a child's chosen sport or event. Verbal encouragement also plays a major role, but avoid going overboard by being too demanding either physically or emotionally.

Kids tend to imitate their parents' basic eating habits (e.g., portion sizes, going back for seconds, foods selected, attitudes, etc.). Statistics show that if one parent is overweight, there is a 40% chance that his/her child will be overweight. If both parents are overweight, the chances go up to 80%! Too often, parents use food as a reward/pacifier, or they use food deprivation as a punishment. It is critical that parents better educate themselves about balanced nutritional foods and their children's eating patterns, replacing a large percentage of the "junk" with healthy substitutes.

The benefits recognized are the same as for adults; improved appearance, easier weight control, better posture and coordination, increased sense of well-being, enhanced relaxation, and overall sound health.

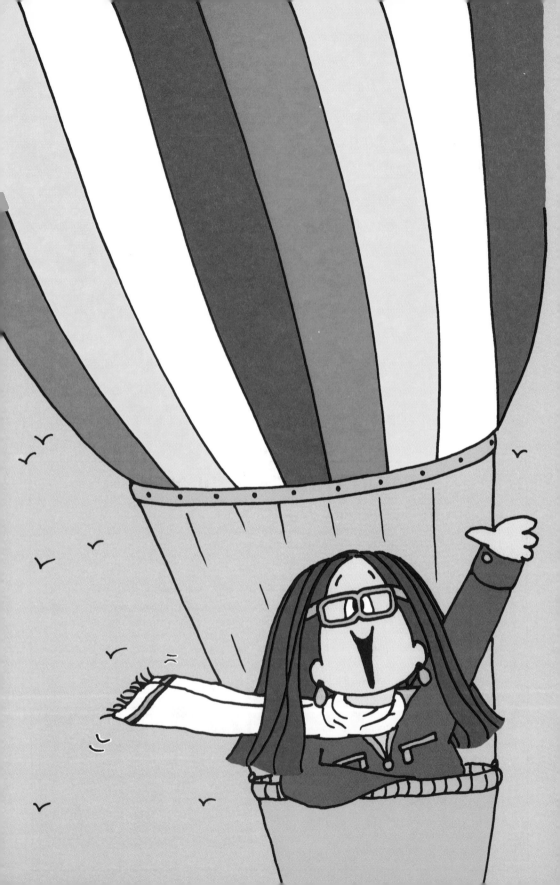

It is the inalienable right
of all to be happy.

- Elizabeth Cady Stanton

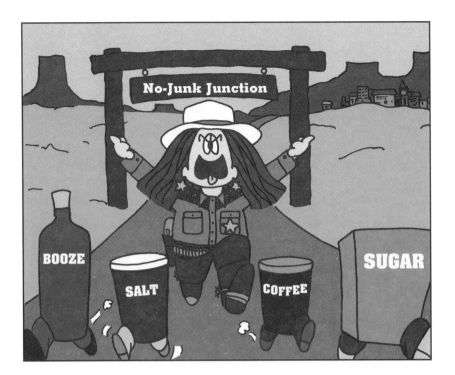

nasty odds & ends

It's time to take a look at a few trouble-makers in the categories of drinking and sprinkling. The same questions are constantly asked regarding table sugar (sucrose), salt (sodium chloride), caffeine, and alcohol, "What effect do they have on my body? How much is too much? How can they be avoided?" Let's take a look at the facts:

SALT

Your body needs sodium, but not much. While one-fifth of a teaspoon daily will keep you healthy, and up to two teaspoons probably won't hurt you, many people average over five teaspoons a day. The sodium that naturally occurs in almost everything we eat typically accounts for about 25% of a person's total intake, and another 25% comes straight out of a shaker. Surprisingly, the remaining 50% is found in packaged and processed foods.

Salt's two biggest crimes are that it may contribute to hypertension and promotes water retention. The best way to cut down on your sodium is to replace salt with other spices and flavorings, and stick to fresh foods in their most natural form.

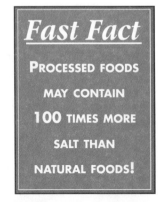

Fast Fact

Processed foods may contain 100 times more salt than natural foods!

ALCOHOL

Booze is definitely not a friend of the trim and healthy! Alcohol's harmful effects on the body are too numerous to list, but here are a few to think about: 1) Provides totally empty calories (and plenty of them) with no nutritive value; 2) Causes liver damage; 3) Decreases your blood's ability to carry oxygen; 4) Impairs judgement, increasing the likelihood of binge/poor eating; and 5) Leads to 50% of all car accidents.

Alcohol is a diuretic and a depressant which should be avoided. If you are going to indulge, keep it to a minimum (especially if you are interested in losing weight) and never substitute alcohol calories for a nutritious meal.

SUGAR

Let's not candy-coat it — large amounts of sugar decays your teeth and makes you fat. However, most people don't realize that eating sugar also has a very harmful effect on blood sugar (glucose) levels. Overly-processed, sugary foods only "give you energy" for a short time; then glucose levels dramatically drop, leaving you feeling hungry and drained. Unfortunately, in this weakened condition people often reach for more sweets.

The average American eats more than two pounds of sugar per week...that's over 3500 calories! 75% of this sugar is "hidden" in foods in the form of additives, preservatives, and a wide variety of sweeteners (e.g., fructose, maltose, dextrose, lactose). In fact, almost all prepared foods have sugar in them. Control your intake by choosing foods in their most unprocessed forms, and keep candies, cakes, and cookies to a minimum.

CAFFEINE

The most common dietary sources of this stimulant drug are coffee, tea, soft drinks, and chocolate. Caffeine temporarily agitates many bodily functions (including heart rate, blood pressure, digestive processes, and general awareness) and extremely heavy consumption has been linked to certain illnesses and disorders.

Coffee is the nation's biggest offender, with approximately 180 milligrams of caffeine in an eight-ounce serving. While teas generally have half as much caffeine as coffee, and sodas even less, these beverages often come in larger portions. Find out about the high acidity and chemical impurities sometimes found in decaffeinated coffees and teas. Cut down your use by substituting low-calorie, healthier alternatives.

POWER SNACKING

We have truly reached the age of the smart snack. There are hundreds of delicious low fat options for anyone willing to take the time to explore. Check out the produce section at your supermarket, or get a little adventurous and visit a market with a reputation for offering natural foods (fruits and vegetables lead the way as traditional favorites). Try replacing potato chips with pretzels, spread jelly on toast instead of butter, eat a bagel rather than a doughnut, and by all means experiment with the endless types of low fat and nonfat frozen yogurt. Get creative...your taste buds and waistline will thank you.

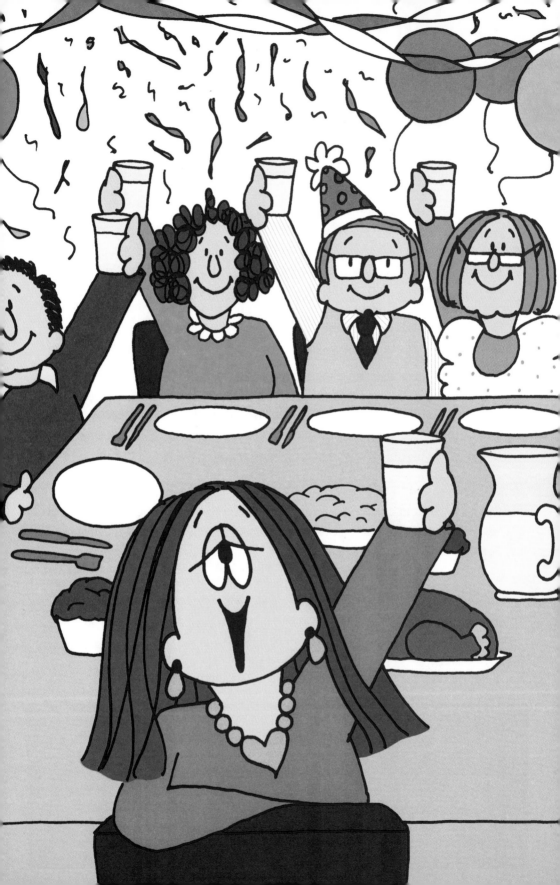

If you can't say you love where you are, what you're doing, and who you're with, ask yourself why and make the necessary adjustments.

- Ramona Cox

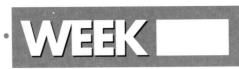

WEEK ☐

MONDAY
- 🍴 ___ *date:* / / *notes:* _____
- ⚖️ ___ _____
- 🏋️ ___ _____
- 🏃 ___ _____

TUESDAY
- 🍴 ___ *date:* / / *notes:* _____
- ⚖️ ___ _____
- 🏋️ ___ _____
- 🏃 ___ _____

WEDNESDAY
- 🍴 ___ *date:* / / *notes:* _____
- ⚖️ ___ _____
- 🏋️ ___ _____
- 🏃 ___ _____

THURSDAY
- 🍴 ___ *date:* / / *notes:* _____
- ⚖️ ___ _____
- 🏋️ ___ _____
- 🏃 ___ _____

FRIDAY
- 🍴 ___ *date:* / / *notes:* _____
- ⚖️ ___ _____
- 🏋️ ___ _____
- 🏃 ___ _____

SATURDAY
- 🍴 ___ *date:* / / *notes:* _____
- ⚖️ ___ _____
- 🏋️ ___ _____
- 🏃 ___ _____

SUNDAY
- 🍴 ___ *date:* / / *notes:* _____
- ⚖️ ___ _____
- 🏋️ ___ _____
- 🏃 ___ _____

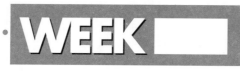
WEEK

MONDAY
___ *date:* / / *notes:* _____
___ _____
___ _____
___ _____

TUESDAY
___ *date:* / / *notes:* _____
___ _____
___ _____
___ _____

WEDNESDAY
___ *date:* / / *notes:* _____
___ _____
___ _____
___ _____

THURSDAY
___ *date:* / / *notes:* _____
___ _____
___ _____
___ _____

FRIDAY
___ *date:* / / *notes:* _____
___ _____
___ _____
___ _____

SATURDAY
___ *date:* / / *notes:* _____
___ _____
___ _____
___ _____

SUNDAY
___ *date:* / / *notes:* _____
___ _____
___ _____
___ _____

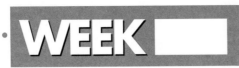

WEEK

MONDAY

date: / / _notes:_

TUESDAY

date: / / _notes:_

WEDNESDAY

date: / / _notes:_

THURSDAY

date: / / _notes:_

FRIDAY

date: / / _notes:_

SATURDAY

date: / / _notes:_

SUNDAY

date: / / _notes:_

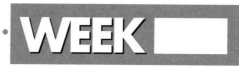
WEEK

MONDAY
___ *date:* / / *notes:* _____
___ _____
___ _____
___ _____

TUESDAY
___ *date:* / / *notes:* _____
___ _____
___ _____
___ _____

WEDNESDAY
___ *date:* / / *notes:* _____
___ _____
___ _____
___ _____

THURSDAY
___ *date:* / / *notes:* _____
___ _____
___ _____
___ _____

FRIDAY
___ *date:* / / *notes:* _____
___ _____
___ _____
___ _____

SATURDAY
___ *date:* / / *notes:* _____
___ _____
___ _____
___ _____

SUNDAY
___ *date:* / / *notes:* _____
___ _____
___ _____
___ _____

WEEK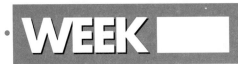

MONDAY

date: / /   notes:

TUESDAY

date: / /   notes:

WEDNESDAY

date: / /   notes:

THURSDAY

date: / /   notes:

FRIDAY

date: / /   notes:

SATURDAY

date: / /   notes:

SUNDAY

date: / /   notes:

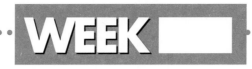
WEEK

MONDAY
___ *date:* / / *notes:* _____
___ _____
___ _____
___ _____

TUESDAY
___ *date:* / / *notes:* _____
___ _____
___ _____
___ _____

WEDNESDAY
___ *date:* / / *notes:* _____
___ _____
___ _____
___ _____

THURSDAY
___ *date:* / / *notes:* _____
___ _____
___ _____
___ _____

FRIDAY
___ *date:* / / *notes:* _____
___ _____
___ _____
___ _____

SATURDAY
___ *date:* / / *notes:* _____
___ _____
___ _____
___ _____

SUNDAY
___ *date:* / / *notes:* _____
___ _____
___ _____
___ _____

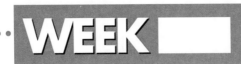
WEEK

MONDAY
date: / / notes:

TUESDAY
date: / / notes:

WEDNESDAY
date: / / notes:

THURSDAY
date: / / notes:

FRIDAY
date: / / notes:

SATURDAY
date: / / notes:

SUNDAY
date: / / notes:

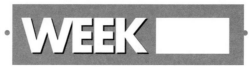

WEEK

MONDAY

____ *date:* / / *notes:* _____
____ _____
____ _____
____ _____

TUESDAY

____ *date:* / / *notes:* _____
____ _____
____ _____
____ _____

WEDNESDAY

____ *date:* / / *notes:* _____
____ _____
____ _____
____ _____

THURSDAY

____ *date:* / / *notes:* _____
____ _____
____ _____
____ _____

FRIDAY

____ *date:* / / *notes:* _____
____ _____
____ _____
____ _____

SATURDAY

____ *date:* / / *notes:* _____
____ _____
____ _____
____ _____

SUNDAY

____ *date:* / / *notes:* _____
____ _____
____ _____
____ _____

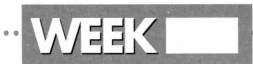
WEEK ⬜

MONDAY
date: / / _notes:_ _____
_____
_____
_____

TUESDAY
date: / / _notes:_ _____
_____
_____
_____

WEDNESDAY
date: / / _notes:_ _____
_____
_____
_____

THURSDAY
date: / / _notes:_ _____
_____
_____
_____

FRIDAY
date: / / _notes:_ _____
_____
_____
_____

SATURDAY
date: / / _notes:_ _____
_____
_____
_____

SUNDAY
date: / / _notes:_ _____
_____
_____
_____

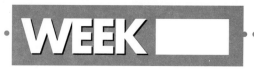

WEEK

MONDAY

date: / / notes:

____
____
____
____

TUESDAY

date: / / notes:

____
____
____
____

WEDNESDAY

date: / / notes:

____
____
____
____

THURSDAY

date: / / notes:

____
____
____
____

FRIDAY

date: / / notes:

____
____
____
____

SATURDAY

date: / / notes:

____
____
____
____

SUNDAY

date: / / notes:

____
____
____
____